Healthy Diet, Happy Bladder

How Diet Affects Bladder Behavior

Elizabeth E. Houser, M.D.

TABLE OF CONTENTS

ACKNOWLEDGEMENTS

I want to thank my husband, Chuck, and my coauthor of the book *A Woman's Guide to Pelvic Health: Expert Advice for Women of All Ages*, Stephanie Hahn, for their unending support and advice.

I also am grateful to Stephanie Yeh, who not only encouraged me to write this book, but guided me through the process.

Lastly, I am grateful to my patients who, over the years, taught me through their experiences that a healthy diet really could lead to a happy bladder.

1. HOW A HEALTHY DIET LEADS TO A HAPPY BLADDER

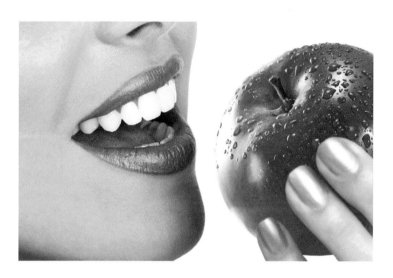

Everywhere we look in the media, we find claims that different diets can improve our quality of life. Experts and gurus suggest that we increase our water intake, avoid sugar, become vegetarian, or try a vegan or gluten-free diet. If we follow the advice of these experts, supposedly our heart, pancreas, and colon will become healthier.

Sadly, very few experts discuss diets that support and promote bladder health. At the same time, with baby boomers continuing to age, bladder problems such as urinary urgency, frequency, and leakage are becoming very common.

Consider these statistics:

➤ One in four women over age 26 experience stress incontinence (urinary leakage when laughing, sneezing, or putting stress on the bladder) at some point in their lives.

➤ About 17% of women in the U.S. suffer from urge incontinence or overactive bladder (urinary urgency, frequency, and leakage).

➤ Some women have both stress and urge incontinence (mixed urinary incontinence), and often have the most severe urinary symptoms.

At the same time, research indicates that diet modifications can be an effective conservative therapy for all three types of urinary incontinence. Believe it or not, what you put in your mouth really can affect the health and behavior of your bladder, especially if you suffer from symptoms of urinary incontinence.

The old adage says, "You are what you eat." For instance, most of us know that spicy peppers can adversely affect our bowels. Just think back to your last case of Montezuma's revenge!

The same saying holds true for bladder health and bladder control. For example, drinking beer can increase the number of trips you make to the bathroom. Why? Because alcohol is a diuretic, which puts the kidneys into overdrive and causes urinary frequency. However, alcohol has a secondary and lesser-known effect on the bladder: alcohol has a direct irritating effect on the bladder lining, which can increase urinary urgency, frequency, and leakage.

It turns out that alcohol is only one of many bladder irritants. In a later section we will discuss various types of bladder irritants. You may be surprised at the number of foods and beverages in your current diet can cause your bladder to overreact.

The good news for those with urinary incontinence is that symptoms can be greatly alleviated by making smart dietary modifications.

Diet modification can include:
- ➢ managing fluid intake
- ➢ avoiding bladder irritants

➤ taking emergency measures as needed

➤ maintaining bowel regularity

These four types of diet modification are neither complicated nor difficult to integrate into your lifestyle. Best of all, these conservative therapies can help you regain bladder control. Read on for the details of each of these therapies.

2. IS YOUR BLADDER HAPPY?

Not sure if your bladder is healthy and happy? Answer the questions in this short quiz to find out.

Check if "Yes"

1. Do you leak urine when you cough, sneeze, or laugh?

   _____

2. Do you feel the sudden urge to urinate whether or not you experience urine leakage?

   _____

3. Do you wake up two or more times per night to urinate?

   _____

4. Do you feel the need to urinate more than eight times per day?

   _____

5. Do you feel the need to urinate shortly after you have just urinated?

   _____

6. Do you leak urine during exercise, when you lift something, or when you change position?

_____

7. Do you leak urine when you hear the sound of running water?

_____

8. Do you experience urinary urgency after drinking small amounts of water?

_____

9. Do you leak urine during sex or feel like you might?

_____

10. Do you feel strong urges to urinate after eating or drinking certain foods or beverages?

_____

YOUR SCORE   _____

If you answered "Yes" to two or more of the above questions then your bladder probably is not all that happy with you. In other words, a score of two or higher means that your bladder health could benefit from the bladder-healthy tips in this book! Need to improve your bladder health? Read on...

3. FLUID MANAGEMENT

Almost everywhere we go, we see people carrying water bottles—bottled water, spring water, power water, and enhanced water. Amazingly enough, water has become a multi-million dollar industry!

Ten years ago, no one would have had trouble choosing from among a huge array of clever water carriers. Today the number of water bottles available—with filtering systems or other features—is dizzying. Hydration is hip! But can overdoing hydration actually be drowning our best efforts to achieve a healthy lifestyle?

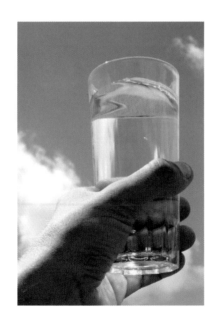

HOW MUCH WATER IS TOO MUCH?

For women with urinary incontinence, figuring out the "right" amount of water to drink can be tricky. How much water is too much water for women coping with urinary incontinence?

The answer is simple: you know you have over-hydrated when your water intake affects your daily activities.

Not sure? Ask yourself these questions:

➢ Do you have to know where the nearest bathroom is on every outing?

➢ Can you sit through a full length film without interruption for a bathroom break?

➢ Do you have to get up more than once at night to urinate?

If you answered "Yes" to any of these questions, then you may need to manage your fluid intake differently. The amount of water intake that is healthy for a person in a 24-hour period varies, depending on a number of lifestyle factors.

HOW MUCH WATER SHOULD YOU DRINK?

Most people need to drink six to eight glasses of water (eight ounces each) in a 24-hour period. For a more customized water-intake figure, follow this rule of thumb:

> *Drink in ounces half your weight in pounds daily.*

For example, if you weigh 150 pounds then, using this formula, you would drink 75 ounces of water per day.

If you exercise, you will need to increase the amount of water you drink to replace the water lost through sweating. Remember also to replace electrolytes.

Another good rule of thumb to determine healthy water intake is to let your thirst be your guide. Drink water when you feel thirsty.

Many people with bladder problems severely limit their water intake, but this action can actually worsen bladder symptoms. Limited water intake tends to concentrate the urine, which can irritate the bladder. Concentrated urine also has a stronger smell than diluted urine, so any urine leakage accidents may be more noticeable. If you have symptoms of urinary incontinence or urgency, don't severely limit the amount of water you drink. Instead, follow the tips given previously to discover your ideal amount of water intake.

Once you have determined the amount of water that is healthy for your weight and lifestyle, consider timing your fluid intake to avoid urinary frequency, urgency, and leakage.

Follow these tips for timing your water intake:

➢ Consume most of your water in the morning.

➢ Avoid too much fluid intake two to three hours before bedtime.

➢ Drink water with a meal rather than in isolation.

THE EFFECT OF WATER ADDITIVES

With so many different kinds of "enhanced" types of water available on the market, women with urinary incontinence symptoms need to pay attention to the actual ingredients in any bottle of water. Many brands of water include a number of additives, some of which can irritate the bladder.

A variety of water products now include added flavors, antioxidants, stimulants, and other ingredients. Since some of these ingredients can irritate the bladder, the best policy is to drink pure water that has no additives. However, if you cannot avoid additive ingredients, try to avoid brands of water that include stimulant additives, such as caffeine, as well as citric flavors. Lemonade and fruit punch powders both contain citric flavoring. When possible, drink pure water with no additives. Tap water is fine to drink, since there is no need to break the bank on bottled water.

4. AVOIDANCE OF BLADDER IRRITANTS

A bladder irritant is any food, beverage, or substance you eat or drink that affects your bladder, causing symptoms such as urinary urgency, frequency, or leakage.

In this section we will discuss not only foods and beverages that can affect your bladder, but also other substances that can have an adverse effect on your bladder. These can include certain food additives, preservatives, and some dietary supplements. Some of these substances directly irritate the bladder, while others are acidic, which lowers the bladder pH and causes bladder spasms.

Common bladder irritants include caffeine, alcohol, citric fruits, and foods containing arylalkylamines (tryptophan, tyrosine, tyramine, and phenylalanine). The toxic effect of some items may not become apparent unless other bladder irritants are present. For instance, your bladder may not react when you eat enchiladas with jalapeno sauce, but add a few margaritas with lime, and you may find your bladder start to spasm. Suddenly the location of the nearest bathroom becomes very important!

CITRIC FOODS AND DRINKS TO AVOID
Many fruits and certain vegetables are acidic, and can cause urinary frequency and urgency. Tomatoes are among the worst offenders. Tomatoes are extremely acidic, and often can be "hidden" ingredients in soups and sauces.

Lemons, limes, oranges, grapefruit, and pineapples are some of the most acidic fruits. In addition, beware of fruit juices, which usually have added sugar and preservatives, both of which may affect the bladder. Low-acid fruits include watermelons, papayas, pears, and apricots.

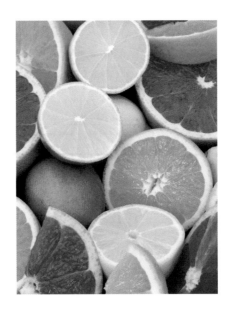

MEAT PRODUCTS AND BLADDER HEALTH

Meat and meat products can also irritate the bladder.

Lean meats are a great source of protein, but they are also a source of acid. All meats and some vegetables contain purines. When your body breaks down purines, the result is uric acid. Your body needs uric acid, the kidneys are responsible for monitoring and regulating the excretion of this acid.

Excess uric acid in the system can lead to health issue such as gout, kidney stones, and gastrointestinal disturbances. Excess acid in the body can lead to intestinal bloating, gas, flatulence, as well as urinary frequency and urgency.

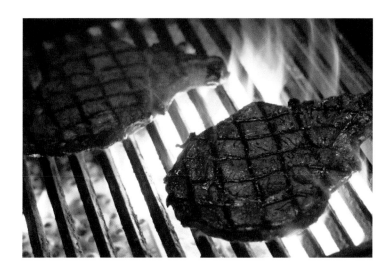

SHOULD YOU GO GLUTEN-FREE?

One of the most popular current dietary guidelines involves avoiding eating wheat, or more specifically, gluten. Although not much has been written about the effects of gluten on the bladder, patients in my practice have seen improvements in their symptoms of bladder irritation when they eat a gluten-free diet.

For these patients, avoiding gluten in their diet, along with other diet changes to reduce bladder irritation resulted in decreased urinary frequency, urgency, and incontinence. Others have noted that avoiding bread that has preservatives, such as BHT and propionic acid, decreased their overactive bladder symptoms.

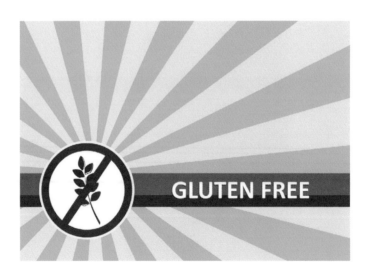

HOW ALCOHOL AFFECTS YOUR BLADDER

Consuming alcohol can negatively affect your bladder in multiple ways.

First, alcohol it is a potent diuretic, which forces your bladder to store more urine. Second, alcohol has a direct irritating effect on the mucosa, or lining, of the bladder. Finally, many alcoholic drinks combine alcohol with other bladder irritants, such as fruit juice and carbonated liquids.

If you do drink alcohol, you can reduce the effects on your bladder by diluting your alcohol intake with water. A good rule of thumb is to drink an eight-ounce glass of water for every alcoholic beverage you consume. While this increased water intake may send you to the bathroom more often, the dilution effect may decrease your chances of having an embarrassing leakage accident!

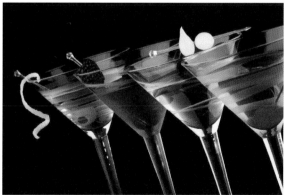

HOW COFFEE AND TEA AFFECT YOUR BLADDER

Both coffee and tea are major bladder irritants because of their caffeine content. Even decaffeinated coffees and teas can irritate your bladder because they still contain some caffeine content.

Caffeine affects your body and bladder in ways similar to alcohol. The diuretic effect causes increased urine production, while the acidic nature of coffee and tea can cause direct bladder irritation.

Herbal teas and coffee substitutes may be good options for some people with urinary incontinence symptoms, while others will need to dilute the effects of caffeine with water, or some other alkalinizing agent (more information in following sections).

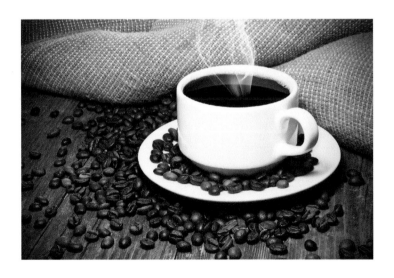

HOW ARTIFICIAL SWEETENERS AND PRESERVATIVES AFFECT YOUR BLADDER

The use of artificial sweeteners in our diets is somewhat controversial in nutrition literature. While these sugar substitutes may help control caloric intake, most nutritionists recommend using natural sweeteners, such as stevia, instead of artificial sweeteners.

Remember the big scare in the 1970s when lab rats developed bladder cancer after being force fed saccharin? Subsequent research on humans showed that artificial sweeteners did not result in increased incidences of bladder cancer. In fact, no studies on human have linked the development of cancer to artificial sweeteners.

However, artificial sweeteners can still irritate the bladder. This is because the body converts certain of these sweeteners during metabolism to sugar alcohols. As already discussed, alcohol is a bladder irritant, and can lead to urinary frequency, urgency, and leakage.

Many food preservatives are also bladder irritants. Benzoic acid, a preservative in many fruit juices and carbonated beverages, is often combined with citric acid to improve flavor. Sulfites, or sulfur dioxide, also acidic in nature, are used in wines, fruits, and vegetables, to preserve color and flavor. When you put any form of "acid" in your body, the result may be an overactive bladder. If you tend to have urinary frequency, urgency, or urgency incontinence, it is wise to avoid any preservative that has a color, number, or initial in its name. Bladder-healthy preservatives include salt, sugar, and rosemary. Read ingredient labels carefully, and remember that the first three ingredients listed are the strongest ingredients in the product.

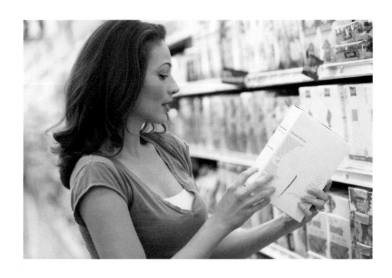

Many ingested substances can irritate the bladder lining, resulting in increased trips to the bathroom and, in some cases, leakage accidents on the way to the bathroom.

You can limit or eliminate some of these ingredients from your diet, minimizing their negative effects. With other ingredients, you may have better luck counteracting their effects with other measures. Read on to learn how to minimize the impact of those dietary items offensive to your bladder.

5. THREE EMERGENCY MEASURES

The word "emergency" may sound a little extreme and urgent, but if you just love margaritas with extra lime plus enchiladas with hot sauce, you will be glad to have the following information on emergency measures.

#1: THE DILUTION STRATEGY

For every irritating beverage (alcohol, caffeine, citric juice) that you imbibe, drink eight ounces of water. The best approach is to alternate the irritating fluid with glasses of water. If you cannot follow this strategy, simply drink several ounces of water when you can.

Keep in mind that what goes in must come out. Plus, most bladder irritants are also diuretics, which will increase urine volume. Add in the glasses of water you drink between other beverages, and you will realize that you may need to visit the bathroom frequently.

The same solution applies to the foods you consume that might irritate the bladder. Dilute the irritants in your urine with water.

#2: USE PRELIEF

There is an over-the-counter supplement that de-acidifies food and drink. The supplement is called *Prelief*, and is made by the same company that makes Beano. It is available in most large drugstore chains. Simply follow the instructions on the bottle. Many of my patients have had considerable success using this simple supplement.

#3: THE BICARBONATE SLUSH

Another "emergency" measure is called the bicarbonate slush. You can make this emergency slush by following this recipe:

Mix one tablespoon baking soda with 16 ounces water.

Stir the mixture thoroughly and drink it right away. Drink eight more ounces of water immediately following the slush. This bicarbonate drink helps neutralize the acidic contents of any offending foods or drinks.

6. MAINTAINING BOWEL REGULARITY

An irritable or constipated colon may result in an irritable bladder. Plus, the constant straining associated with constipation can often make symptoms of urinary incontinence worse. Most people know that increasing fluid intake and fiber helps combat chronic constipation.

Many "natural" fiber additives are also available on the market. Some familiar brands include *Metamucil* and *Citrucel*. Be aware that if you use any of these fiber supplements, you will need to increase your water intake.

Miralax is an osmotic laxative, meaning that it draws fluid from the body into the colon to promote normal bowel movements. Now available over the counter, this supplement is safe to use daily. It is tasteless and less grainy than any other fiber supplements. Another benefit of this supplement is that it dissolves easily when stirred into water, juice, or coffee.

To alleviate chronic constipation, try to avoid laxatives that produce cramping and watery diarrhea. Examples of these kinds of laxatives include *Dulcolax* and *Ex-Lax*. In dire situations,

Fleet enemas are the better option. These enemas are easy to self-administer and safe to use.

FLAX SEED FOR BOWEL REGULARITY
Flax seed is a very popular supplement for maintaining bowel regularity, with good reason.

Flax seed contains three components responsible for its health benefits:

- ➢ omega-3 essential fatty acides
- ➢ lignans
- ➢ fiber

Omega-3 essential fatty acids have been shown to have heart benefits. Each tablespoon of ground flax seed has about 1.8 grams of omega-3s.

Lignans, found in flax seed, are antioxidants and contain plant estrogen. The concentration of lignans in flax seed is much higher than in other plant sources.

Finally, flax seed is a great source of fiber. For constipation, use this recipe:

Add ¼ cup of freshly ground flax seed to eight ounces cold juice or water.

You can use an inexpensive coffee grinder, dedicated to grinding flax seed, and grind the seeds fresh daily. You can also grind your flax seed less often and store it in the refrigerator in a sealed bag.

However, note that if you grind your flax seed less frequently, you will lose some of the health benefits. When ground well, flax see has a nutty flavor that is not unpleasant once you become accustomed.

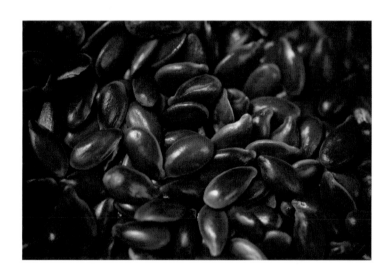

PRESCRIPTION MEDICATIONS AND CONSTIPATION

It is worthwhile to discuss how certain prescription medications can affect bowel function. Many prescription medications have anti-cholenergic effects on the bowel. This means that they inhibit the cholinergic receptors that are responsible for normal bowel motility.

Other medications may have other effects on the colon that could produce constipation. When your doctor or other healthcare provider starts you on a new medication, be sure to ask if constipation is a common side effect. If so, ask for tips you can use to offset that effect.

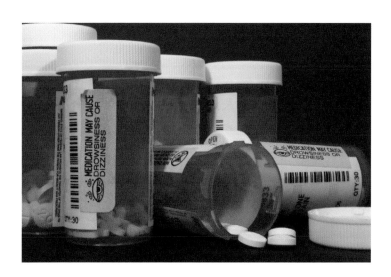

SUPPLEMENTS AND CONSTIPATION

Some supplements, especially calcium, can be very constipating.

Many women over 50—and there are millions of us—are told to take calcium supplements religiously to prevent or minimize osteoporosis.

Recognizing this fact, and that many women will discontinue calcium supplementation because of constipation, companies have started adding components to calcium supplements to offset the constipating effects.

Many products on the market combine fiber with calcium. These include *Fiber Choice with Calcium*, *Metamucil Strong Bones*, and *Citrucel Soft Chews with Calcium*, to name a few. Ask your pharmacist which might best suit your needs.

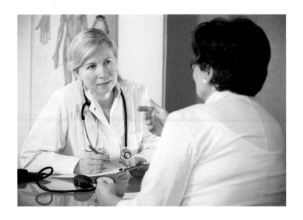

Magnesium is often taken with calcium to mitigate constipation. Calcium/magnesium supplements are available in liquid, chewable, and capsule form. You can also combine the two supplements yourself simply by taking calcium supplements along with magnesium supplements.

Make it a goal to prevent severe constipation by the use any of the measures discussed above. In addition, always discuss with your doctor any bowel irregularities that last over 7 to 10 days.

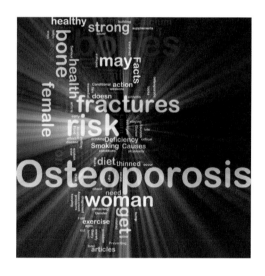

7. AT THE END OF THE DAY

We really are what we eat and drink. Our dietary intake affects the heart, colon, organs, and skin.

More importantly, for those with urinary incontinence or bladder issues, diet affects the bladder. Some people are affected more than others.

Urinary frequency, urgency and incontinence **can** be minimized or avoided if your bladder is sensitive to your diet. Use the information in this book to make educated choices about what you put in your mouth.

A healthy diet leads to a healthy you... and a happy bladder!

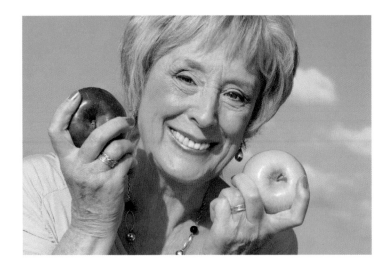

8. RESOURCES

Want to know more about bladder and pelvic health? The following resources are wonderful educational resources on these topics:

A Woman's Guide to Pelvic Health: Expert Advice for Women of All Ages
By Elizabeth E. Houser, M.D. and Stephanie Riley Hahn, P.T.
(available at Amazon, Barnes & Noble, and major booksellers)

A Woman's Guide to Pelvic Health online
➢ Website: www.AWomansGuidetoPelvicHealth.com
➢ Blog: www.AWomansGuidetoPelvicHealth.com/blog
➢ Ebook: www.AWomansGuidetoPelvicHealth.com/ebook
➢ YouTube: www.YouTube.com/user/wetmatters
➢ Facebook: www.facebook.com/awomansguidetopelvichealth
➢ Twitter: twitter.com/pelvic_health

American Academy of Family Physicians
P.O. Box 11210
Shawnee Mission, KS 66207-1210
800-274-2237 or 913-906-6000
www.aafp.org/afp/20000701/127.html

American Association of Sexuality Educators,
Counselors and Therapists
P.O. Box 1960
Ashland, VA 23005
804-752-0026
www.aasect.org

American College of Obstetricians and
Gynecologists – (search for "Urinary
incontinence")
P.O. Box 96920
409 12th Street SW
Washington, DC 20090-6920
202-863-2518
www.acog.org

American Physical Therapy Association
Section on Women's Health
P.O. Box 327
Alexandria, VA 22313
800-999-APTA, ext. 3229
www.womenshealthapta.org

American Urological Association Foundation
1000 Corporate Boulevard
Linthicum, MD 21090
1-866-746-4282 (toll free, U.S. only)
www.urologyhealth.org

Medline Plus
National Library of Medicine
8600 Rockville Pike
Bethesda, MD 20894
1-888-FIND-NLM or 301-594-5983
www.nlm.nih.gov/medlineplus/femalesexualdysfunction.html
www.nlm.nih.gov/medlineplus/urinaryincontinence.html

National Association for Continence
P.O. Box 1019
Charleston, SC 29402-1019
1-800-BLADDER or 843-377-0900
www.nafc.org/media/media-kit/facts-statistics

National Institutes of Health State-of-the-Science
Conference Statement:
Prevention of Fecal and Urinary Incontinence in
Adults, Annals of Internal Medicine
www.annals.org/cgi/content/full/148/6/449

National Kidney and Urologic Diseases
Clearinghouse
3 Information Way
Bethesda, MD 20892-3580
1-800-891-5390
www.kidney.niddk.nih.gov/Kudiseases/pubs/uiw
omen/index.htm

North American Menopause Society
5900 Landerbrook Drive, Suite 390
Mayfield Heights, OH 44124
440-442-7550
www.menopause.org

Sexuality Information and Education Council of
the United States
90 John Street, Suite 704
New York, NY 10038
212-819-9770
www.siecus.org

Society for Sex Therapy and Research
409 12th Street SW
Washington, DC 20090-6920
202-863-1648
www.sstarnet.org

Society for the Scientific Study of Sexuality
P.O. Box 416
Allentown, PA 18105-0416
610-443-3100
www.sexscience.org

UroToday
1802 Fifth Street
Berkeley, CA 94710
510-540-0930 (fax)
info@urotoday.com
www.urotoday.com/stress-urinary-incontinence-1483.html

9. ABOUT
ELIZABETH E. HOUSER, M.D.

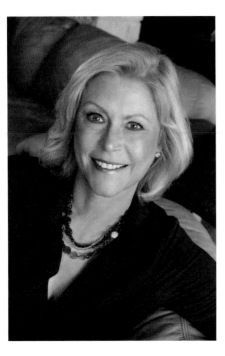

Dr. Houser is a board certified urologist who practiced urology in Austin, Texas for many years. She now works as an author, pelvic floor consultant, and Pilates instructor.

She graduated in 1987 from the University of Texas Health Science Center at San Antonio Medical School, and completed her residency in urology at the same facility in 1993.

Her media appearances include *The Today Show*, *KXAN*, *KEYE*, and *KVUE*. She coauthored the book *A Woman's Guide to Pelvic Health: Expert Advice for Women of All Ages*, published by John Hopkins University Press in 2012 (www.AWomansGuideToPelvicHealth.com). She has authored several chapters in medical texts and handbooks, as well as articles in scientific journals.

Recently Dr. Houser was a featured speaker at the *Texas Women in Business Wellness Fair* in Austin, Texas, and was featured in *Austin Woman* magazine in March, 2013. She has written several articles for national magazines, and has served as a guest blogger.

In her Pilates practice Dr. Houser hopes to help women with pelvic floor problems through Pilates-based exercise.

She lives in Austin with her husband, Chuck, and Jack Russell terrier, Bud.

Printed in Poland
by Amazon Fulfillment
Poland Sp. z o.o., Wrocław

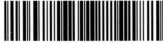
49930820R00026